10 Lies Your Herbalist Told You

LISA BARGER

WHO I AM & WHY I WROTE THIS BOOK

My name is Lisa Barger. I am a master herbalist and have spent the past twenty years sharing what I know about herbs and herbal remedies, essential oils and "alternative" therapies like Tai Chi, acupuncture and more. Name a major branch of "natural" health; I've probably studied it.

I am the founder of, and principle writer for, a network of websites covering everything from herbal remedies to child safety to pet food recalls. I cover the good and the bad of natural health—and expose the bogus.

I'm also the author of several books. I wrote books like *Coffee, Tea & Water, Alt Med & Sexual Health* and *An Historical Look at Bach Flower Remedies.*

But from even my earliest days studying herbs and folk remedies I also realized there was a lot of room for charlatans, quacks and scammers. And I saw firsthand how few of my fellow "natural" practitioners were willing to speak up and hold those cheaters accountable.

So I did.

It soon became clear I no longer belonged in "natural medicine"—and perhaps never had. I took the words "naturopath" an "herbalist" off my business cards and focused on covering alternative medicine news.

10 Lies Your Herbalist Told You is a small collection of natural health myths I've debunked over the years. My hope is that these essays will help you find the information you need to make an informed choice about your own health. There's a **lot** of bad information floating around out there. I hope this book does just a bit to make the scams easier to spot.

"It's YOUR health. Don't leave it up to someone else." ~ Lisa Barger

CONTENTS

THIS BOOKLET WAS PREVIOUSLY PUBLISHED

10 Lies Your Herbalist Told You is composed of Q&As, essays and news articles that were previously published in other formats, including websites, newsletters and syndicated news columns.

THIS BOOKLET IS NOT A MEDICAL TEXT

10 Lies Your Herbalist Told You is not a medical text; nothing in this booklet is presented as medical advice.

It is not the author's intention to encourage self-diagnosis or self-treatment.

ABOUT THIS BOOKLET'S REFERENCES

This booklet was written for the natural health enthusiasts who cannot be satisfied with vague "they say" and "studies prove" claims. In that spirit, the author has chosen a streamlined format for *10 Lies Your Herbalist Told You*'s references

FINANCIAL DISCLOSURE

Neither Lisa Barger nor anyone associated with the LisaBarger.com family of websites has any financial relationship with any person or business mentioned in this text.

Lisa Barger has no relationship with, or "rep" for, any multi-level-marketing (MLM) firm, pharmaceutical company or herbal remedies business.

"JOHN WAYNE DIED WITH 40 POUNDS OF FECES IN HIS GUT."

The complete and utter lie about John Wayne and how he died with "40 to 60 pounds" of something called "intestinal buildup" in his colon was one of the first herbal medicine myths I ever debunked.

The story varies, according to which scammy website you're reading, but it usually goes something like this:

"The average American carries around pounds and pounds of rotting fecal matter in his colon. John Wayne's autopsy found 40 pounds of decaying fecal matter in his gut. Elvis had 60 pounds of excess fecal matter in him when he died."

Oftentimes the story cites a 1999 *USA Today* article that "proves" the John Wayne story is true and includes warnings about how we get these "mucoid plaques" and "old fecal buildups" because here in America we eat so much junk food. Naturally, the only way to get rid of all those "toxins" is to use some sort of "colon cleansing" program--some of which cost hundreds of dollars.

The truth, though, is that it's all a complete and utter lie:

- First of all, John Wayne did not die of colon cancer, as some versions of this story claim—he actually died of stomach cancer. Furthermore, Wayne reportedly had surgery to remove a tumor from his intestines just a few weeks before he died. Surely if he'd had a 40-pound mass of rotting fecal matter in his colon his doctors would have (a) found it and (b) removed it.

1

- Second, even if the story about him having all that fecal matter in his gut was true we would never have known it because Wayne was never autopsied. There was no mystery about how he died so there was no need for an autopsy. There's absolutely no evidence that anyone ever removed and weighed his internal organs.

- Third, the *USA Today* story doesn't actually exist--at least not as it's claimed in the myth.

So why would someone spread such a lie? And why would they attach such famous names to it? And why would they continue to spread those lies even after the lies were so completely exposed as false?

I think we all know the answer to that--to sell you something. And what they want to sell you is the topic of our next myth . . .

"YOUR GUT IS FULL OF 'MUCOID PLAQUE' & OLD FECES."

You've never heard of mucoid plaque? Don't worry. As I said in one of the first pieces I ever wrote on mucoid plaque, it's completely bogus. Here's that article:

Mucoid Plaque

You can hardly turn on your television without being bombarded with informercials for "natural" colon cleansers. But are herbal-based colon cleansers really effective or are they just another attempt to sell you another "natural" product that you don't really need? Here's the truth about these "natural" cleansing products—from someone who has devoted her career to the study of natural medicine:

Where Did The Idea Of Colon Cleansing Come From?

Colon cleansing is a very old therapy that goes back to at least the ancient Egyptians. They believed that all disease started out as rotting food in the bowel and wrote extensively about various ways to rid the body of this "poison". Modern science has completely disproved this idea but for some reason, many in "natural" medicine just won't let it go. Then, a few years ago, the "rotting food in the bowel" idea found a new audience, thanks in large part to internet discussion groups.

Not only do many "natural" practitioners embrace this discredited idea, they go even further by claiming that we're all going through life with 5 to

45 pounds of old, impacted feces inside our guts. And, as you've probably seen, some of them have produced some pretty explicit photos to back up their stories.

But Mucoid Plaque Is A Complete & Utter Myth

On some infomercials (and several web sites) you'll see the term "mucoid plaque". This is the mucous-based "stuff", for lack of a better term, that's supposedly coating the inside of your colon and preventing your large intestine from working properly. The truth is, mucoid plaque doesn't even exist.

The term "mucoid plaque" is a term created by a writer named Richard Anderson who—and this will come as no surprise to the skeptics—sells colon cleansers. And Anderson even acknowledges making up the term in his article, "What Is Mucoid Plaque". The phrase does not appear in any medical text—only this article.

So Why Do People Think Colon Cleansers Work?

To fully understand how cleansers trick people into believing that they work, it's important to explain exactly what they are. And what the vast majority of herbal-based colon cleaners are, is just plain old fiber. Now, some have herbs and other ingredients with believed anti-parasitic and/or laxative properties, but colon cleansers are mainly just fiber. And fiber "bulks up" when it comes into contact with moisture. In fact, you can demonstrate this yourself by dropping a capsule into water and watching how it expands as the shell dissolves.

So let's assume that you're a typical American. You probably eat a diet that's relatively low in raw fruits, fresh vegetables and whole grains. In other words, you probably have a diet that's pretty low in fiber. And you probably have only a few bowel movements a week.

But let's say that you begin a cleansing regimen. Your dietary fiber probably doubles (or even triples) and you now have 2 or 3 bowel movements a day for 2 or 3 days in a row. Maybe your bowel movements are more comfortable and, maybe, when you "go", you feel "finished" for the first time in a very long time. That's exactly what fiber does—it speeds up your colon, bulks up your stool, and helps some people feel "empty" after they use the toilet.

Now, isn't it easy to understand why so many people feel that they're being "cleaned out" when they use a colon cleanser? After all, what could possibly be wrong with bigger, more frequent and vastly more comfortable bowel movements?

Is Colon Cleansing Harmful?

The truth is, most colon cleansers are probably perfectly harmless. But you can get exactly the same effect just by consuming plain old psyllium—the "active" ingredient in Metamucil®—for far less money. Whether you decide to do a colon cleanse or not is entirely up to you. Many people find that a colon cleanse is a great kick-start to a new, healthier eating regimen. But if you decide to pass, that's OK, too.

And Here's My Best Argument Against Colon Cleansers:

Have you ever had a colonoscopy? If you have, then you know that in the days leading up to your procedure, your doctor has you follow a fairly strict regimen of food and drugs to empty your colon. Yet, no one doing this type of cleanse ever reports passing black, rubbery bowel movements like the ones you see on colon cleansing web sites. And if you've ever accompanied your partner to his or her colonoscopy, you know that all the doctor sees is pink, clean tissue.

Where did all the "dried up" or "excess" fecal matter go? It wasn't voided during the pre-operative cleanse and it doesn't show up on camera during the procedure. Thousands of colonoscopies are performed every year in this country but not a single one has ever found evidence that we're all walking around with "dried up" fecal matter just waiting to make us sick.

####

That wasn't my only attempt to debunk the myth of "mucoid plaque". I followed that one with an article I wrote back in 2008 titled "*What is Mucoid Plaque?*"

What Is Mucoid Plaque?

Mucoid plaque is an imaginary toxin that some "natural" practitioners and most colon cleansing companies claim we all have inside our large intestines. It was apparently coined by a self-described naturopath named Richard Anderson, who authored the *Cleanse & Purify Thyself* series of books.

The truth is, "mucoid plaque" is a made-up phrase that is most often used to scare you into buying an expensive and unnecessary herbal colon cleanser. The man who claims to have coined the phrase has never been a licensed physician but instead claims to have gotten all this new information about colon health from a "divine being". The term "mucoid plaque" doesn't appear in any medical dictionary and even "natural" experts like Dr. Andrew Weil are skeptical.

To help you better understand why mucoid plaque is neither a real medical issue or anything you need to worry about, ask yourself these questions:

- Your entire digestive tract is coated in mucous. If this mucous could truly form hardened, coating "plaques" why don't we see it in other areas of the digestive tract? And how is the mucous in your colon any more dangerous than the mucous, say, in your nose?
- If mucoid plaque is real, why is Anderson the only person to have ever identified it? And why doesn't it show up in autopsies or medical exams like colonoscopies?
- Why is "mucoid plaque" only passed by people using herbal or "natural" colon cleansers? Why don't people who use pre-colonoscopy cleansers like Fleet®—or even just plain old laxatives—ever pass those long, black ropes of feces?

When you look at all the facts, it's easy to see that mucoid plaque is just another one of those terms that has a kernel of truth inside a great big wad of nonsense that's intended to sell you yet another "natural" product you don't really need.

References:

Anderson, R. (1998). Cleanse & Purify Thyself.

Weil, A. (2007). Sea-Salt Flush: What's the Best Cleansing Regime? Retrieved from drweil.com/drw/u/QAA400277/sea-salt-flush on December 10, 2008.

####

Now, of course, once you've made up a scary sounding disease like "mucoid plaque" you need a way to make money from it. I took a look at some of the most common colon cleansing claims in 2010 in my piece "Top 5 Benefits of Colon Cleansing--Is It True?" Here's that article:

Top 5 Benefits of Colon Cleansing--Is It True?

I often get asked why I write so many colon cleansing articles. Here's my answer: There are thousands and thousands of websites, blogs and forum postings out there trying to sell you a product you don't need—and they're using half-truths (and sometimes outright lies) to do it.

Ever see one of those "Top 5" lists for why colon cleansing is so vital to your health? I do—nearly every day—and there's about one kernel of truth in them twisted up in a whole bunch of nonsense and a whole lot of fear-mongering.

Let's look at the top five "benefits" of colon cleansing and break them down one by one:.

Benefit #1: Colon cleansing removes toxic mucoid plaque.

Folks who cite this as a reason to "cleanse" say that cleansing removes a made-up toxic layer known as mucoid plaque. If this "plaque" coating isn't removed, they claim, it sits there in your colon, re-releasing those "toxins". The "toxins" are then re-absorbed into the blood stream and you're less healthy for it.

Truth: "Mucoid plaque" is a made-up phrase that never existed until a guy named Richard Anderson wrote about it in a book about 20 years ago. (Anderson, naturally, formulates a line of "cleansing" products that he'll happily sell you.) But no legitimate medical study—not even one appearing in one of the "alternative" medical journals—has ever documented the existence of this supposedly invisible toxic coating of plaque and the term does not appear in any medical text book we can find.

Benefit #2: Colon cleansing increases your absorption of nutrients.

By removing that toxic layer of gunk, say the sellers of colon cleansers, you increase your absorption of nutrients.

Truth: To understand why this one is false, think back to what you learned in school about digestion. Most of it takes place in the small intestine—not the colon. The colon is capable of absorbing some nutrients but it lacks the special mini-organs known as villi. Those are found only in the small intestine and they are the parts of the digestive system responsible for digestion—not the colon.

Benefit #3: Colon cleansing helps you lose weight.

Cleanse your colon and you can lose 45 pounds some folks say. Some claim it's pounds of "impacted" fecal matter and some claim you'll lose actual body fat.

Truth: You may lose weight during a cleanse but it's a false weight loss because much of what you'll have lost was actually gained after you started the cleanse. Here's why: most of those cleansers (the vast majority of them, in fact) are nearly all fiber. And what does fiber do in your colon? It absorbs water and holds on to it—and it can hold on to a lot. Your first bowel movement after starting a cleanse might result in a 1 or even 2 pound "loss" but it's not fat—it's simply the ingredients of the cleanser and all the moisture they're holding onto.

Benefit #4: Colon cleansing prevents cancer.

Truth: There is some evidence to suggest that a diet rich in fiber may help reduce the risks of certain cancers—including colon cancer—but the exact mechanism by which this happens isn't clear. Some of the early studies on fiber and colon cancer have been criticized for their poor design and some medical experts have theorized that it's not so much the fiber as the antioxidants and other nutrients that high-fiber foods like raw fruits and fresh vegetables offer that's really reducing the risk of cancer.

What no legitimate medical expert believes, though, is that any colon cleanser prevents colon cancer by using fiber to "scrape off" microscopic tumors before they get a chance to become deadly. There's just absolutely no proof whatsoever that that's even possible.

Benefit #5: Colon cleansing speeds up your digestive tract and regulates your bowel movements.

Truth: As with most health myths we tackle here at LisaBarger.com, this one has a kernel of truth to it. Unfortunately for the scam artists, though, it doesn't work quite the way colon cleanser sellers claim. A colon cleaner may increase the number of eliminations you experience per day and it may lower what's call the "transit" time of digested food. But, again, that's the fiber working. You'd get exactly the same effect if you simply added more fiber to your diet.

On the other hand, if you're taking a colon cleanser that contains turkey rhubarb, walnut hulls or cascara, you may very well find that your bowel movements "speed up" as though you'd taken a laxative from the pharmacy department of your local supermarket. And do you want to know why? Those ingredients (and others) act very much like commercial laxatives. The herbs your cleanser contains may be "natural" but they still act by irritating the lining of your colon and cause your colon to "purge" itself—exactly the same way many drugstore laxatives do.

Whether you buy a colon cleanser or not is up to you. My only hope is that I've given you a little information to help you make an informed decision.

Of course, not every scammer pushing the 40-pounds-of-feces myth is hawking herbs. Some would rather sell you on a fancy medical procedure known as colonic irrigation. Check out this piece I wrote on colonic therapy:

Is Colonics Safe?

In response to one of my first-ever articles on alternative medicine, a reader asked, "I read your piece on colonics and I have to say, I don't get why anyone would do this. Is colonics even safe?" My answer was that colonic irrigation is a valid medical procedure but there's nothing "natural" about it.

And it's often not performed legally.

What Colonics Is

When you go in for a colonics treatment, a technician will insert a soft nozzle into your rectum and then force liquid into your large intestine, which is what doctors call your colon. (Hence the terms "colonics" and "colonic hydrotherapy".)

In most cases, you'll be asked to "hold" in the liquid while the technician "massages" your abdominal area—supposedly to "release" stuck feces.

Then, either on your own or with the help of the colonics machine, your colon is allowed to empty itself of the liquid and you're done.

Coffee or Tea, Anyone?

Often, the liquid used is just plain water but some colonics providers use herbal teas or even just plain old coffee. And, yes, you will absorb the caffeine through your colon wall. (Absorbing water is your colon's main function, after all.)

What Colonics Is Supposed to Do for You

Like most people who work in "natural" health, colonics providers believe that the health of your colon is directly tied to the health of the rest of your body. This comes from a very, very old idea that seems to have found new life lately.

Is there any truth to that idea? As a matter of fact, yes. Your intestines are a vital part of your immune system and numerous studies have found that by manipulating the bacterial colonies in your intestinal tract, you may actually be able to reduce symptoms of IBS, allergies and even some types of arthritis.

BUT, colonics themselves are of no known benefit and may be harmful. In 2003, the Attorney General of Texas (where naturopathy is actually illegal and colonics can only be performed under the supervision of a qualified medical physician) sued 6 colonics practitioners after one patient died and several others experienced infections and perforated bowels.

You Tell Me. Is Colonics Safe?

So, after learning the facts about colonics, you tell me. Is this something you would do? Do YOU consider colonics natural?

####

The world of alternative medicine and "natural" health has changed a lot since I wrote those first articles debunking the myths of "mucoid plaque". Back then I was called a "Joe Nobody" by one of the big colon cleanse sellers and labeled a quack.

Today, though, there seem to be fewer of the worst claims being made. I still see photos of people holding up those long, dark "ropes" of feces but I hardly see anyone claiming that we're all walking around with 40 pounds of feces stuck to our insides.

"EAR CANDLES PULL 'TOXINS' FROM YOUR BODY THROUGH YOUR EARS."

Another practice you don't hear much about today is ear candling. Here's one of my earliest pieces on this little bit of quackery:

Ear Candling - A Q&A

Question: *"I read your piece on ear candles and I must say I found it extremely [closed minded]. How do you explain all the studies proving they work?"*

My Answer: I'm not aware of any peer-reviewed studies proving that ear candles remove ear wax, cure inner ear infections or "detox" you. I did, however, find a few reports of people being injured by hot, dripping wax while using the candles.

What Ear Candles Are

Ear candles—just in case you're not familiar with them—are long strips of "natural" fabric (most often linen) that are dipped in melted beeswax then rolled into a hollow cone shape and allowed to harden.

After they harden, ear candles are inserted into the ear canal, lit on fire and allowed to burn down.

Ear candles are supposed to do a variety of things—remove ear wax, reduce ear infections, and increase your lymph flow.

Some Questions to Ask Yourself about Ear Candles

You don't need me to tell you that the "wax" in your ears is extremely sticky—not to mention very thick. How in the world can a "vacuum" created by a small flame possibly be strong enough to "pull" that wax out of your ear canal? And, assuming that it could, how could that "vacuum" not damage your eardrum in the process?

When you stop to think about it, it just doesn't make sense, does it?

So Why Do Ear Candles Work?

You know, I've read a lot of stories about ear candles on the internet but I've never actually met anyone who reported good results from ear candling—except for people selling them.

But let's be fair. Perhaps some people find the process relaxing. (After all, when's the last time you got to lie down and do nothing for 10 minutes in the middle of the day?) If ear candles work for some people, I suspect that the placebo response is at work.

Can Ear Candles Be Dangerous?

Studies show that ear candles don't produce a vacuum or remove ear wax. Furthermore, a few people have actually had their eardrums damaged by wax that dripped into their ears and hardened there.

And don't believe people who tell you that doctors don't like ear candles just because they cut into a doctor's "bottom line", either. The standard treatment for excessive ear wax is an over-the-counter ear wash formula you can buy in any pharmacy and most supermarkets. Doctors have nothing to gain by debunking ear candles.

But, it's your health. Is ear candling something YOU would consider?

References:

Seely, D., et al. (1996). Ear candles—efficacy and safety.

Ernst, E. (2004). Ear candles: a triumph of ignorance over science.

Weil, A. (2005). Melting Out Ear Wax? Q & A Library, DrWeil.com.

Alternative medicine isn't just hawked by medical charlatans. In the early 2000s the internet saw an explosion in the number of made-for-clicks websites. The general idea of these websites (many of which were actually blogs) was that you could choose a topic, throw up a few dozen "articles", put some advertisements on them and make a little extra money. Didn't want to mess with your own website? Dozens and dozens of "content farms" popped up that would take your writings and give you a tiny cut of the ad revenue they made.

Unfortunately, the information on those sites was often written by people with no medical training at all. To call some of that information "questionable" would be generous. And every now and then I'd run across something that actually seemed to advocate something dangerous.

Between 2008 and 2010 a good chunk of my own writing was devoted to answering some of that bad information. This next piece is from 2009 and talks about an article on ear candling in which the author didn't even know what "yeast" was:

Can Ear Candling Remove Candida? - A Q&A

The question: *"I saw [an article on another website] and thought it was interesting. Do you think it's true? Can using ear candles really remove candida bacteria from your body?"*

My answer: First, let's clear up something about the source article— *Candida* is most certainly not a bacterium. I thought the author of that blog had just misspoken until I found a second reference to "candida bacteria" in another of her articles. I mean no offense to the writer, but if she doesn't know the difference between a fungus and a bacterium … already, we're off on the wrong foot.

When people talk about "having candida" they're really talking about an overgrowth of a yeast-like fungus in the *Candida* genus. *Candida albicans* is the most common and is the one most often responsible for the condition most of us call a "yeast infection".

But let's get back to the question … Can ear candling reduce *Candida*? In my opinion, no. I see absolutely no way ear candles can "pull" germs, toxins or anything else from the body. As I stated years ago in my original ear candling article, there is no "gentle vacuum" produced by ear candles and if there was a vacuum strong enough to pull out wax, germs and dirt it would be so strong that it would damage your eardrum.

So, my answer is, "No." There is simply no proof that ear candles do anything even remotely related to "pulling" *Candida* from the body.

References:

Prince, D. (2009). Can Ear Candling Remove Candida? Retrieved from www.healthniche.ca February 25, 2009.

In 2010 the US Food and Drug Administration, or FDA, began to crack down on ear candles and sent official warning letters to several sellers and manufacturers of the quack devices. That, of course, didn't sit well with the people who make, sell and use ear candles so some of them organized an online petition to force the FDA to rethink its position. Here's my piece on that effort:

Ear Candles, FDA & Freedom of Speech

Natural health expert Andrew Weil calls them "hocus pocus" and former UK homeopath Edzard Ernst calls them a "triumph of ignorance". We're talking about ear candles and it seems that the FDA has finally taken a heavier hand in dealing with these quack devices and the people who make and sell them.

Back in February the U.S. Food and Drug Administration, or FDA, sent official Warning Letters to a number of folks who sell ear candles and now, those sellers are striking back.

But instead of defending the medical legitimacy of their ridiculous quackery they're taking an entirely different route.

They want you to sign an online petition. And they're claiming freedom of speech as their main defense.

The organizers of the online petition to overturn the FDA's "ban" on ear candles cite, in part, Justice O'Connor's statement about the "dissemination of truthful information" in the case of Thompson v. Western States Medical Center (535 U.S. 357, 2002).

Now, we're not attorneys (obviously) but one big problem here is the "truthful information" being passed along by manufacturers and sellers of ear candles. We're not sure where the "truthful" information they reference comes from. After all, many of these sellers were, until very recently, still claiming that ear candles "pull" out excess ear wax and remove unnamed "toxins". And there's simply never been any scientific proof that ear candles do any such thing.

So we ask you … what do YOU think? Are the sellers and manufacturers of ear candles really asking President Obama and FDA Commissioner Hamburg to turn a blind eye to devices that have never been proven to work as their proponents claim but which have been linked to a handful of documented injuries? In the name of Free Speech?

Sources:

U.S. Food and Drug Administration. (2010). 2010 Warning Letters accessed April 1, 2010 from fad.gov/.

Natural Solutions Foundation. (2010). Petition accessed April 1, 2010 from salsa.democracyinaction.org.

Ernst, E. (2004). Ear candles: a triumph of ignorance over science. *The Journal of Laryngology and Otology.*

Weil, A. (2005). Melting Out Ear Wax? Q & A Library, DrWeil.com.

####

One of the best pieces I ever saw on ear candles came from Bobby Nelson, writing for the James Randi Educational Foundation website. In that piece Nelson burns 2 sets of ear candles--one in his ears and one in a cardboard box. When the ear candles were cut open and examined post-use, all the candles showed exactly the same "gunk" in them.

This, says Nelson, proves that the "wax" people find in their spent ear candles doesn't come from your ear—and it isn't ear wax. It's simply the beeswax that's already in the candles.

You can see that article here: http://www.randi.org/site/index.php/swift-blog/1265-toss-out-the-q-tips-bring-in-the-ear-candles.html)

"A FAMOUS SINGER GOT CANCER FROM PLASTIC WATER BOTTLES."

This one isn't so much a lie you're told by herbalists or naturopaths, specifically, but it is an urban legend I still see on natural health blogs once in a while. It has to do with the singer Sheryl Crow and how she supposedly got breast cancer from plastic water bottles. The myth goes something like this:

"Sheryl Crow was on the Ellen show and said her doctor told her not to drink water from any plastic bottles that had been left in a hot car. The doctor said that those bottles leach chemicals when they get hot and those toxins are what gave Sheryl breast cancer."

As with all good urban myths, the "facts" change a little bit from telling to telling but that's the general idea--leave a bottle of water in a hot car and cancer-causing chemicals from the bottle leach into the water.

So is any of it true?

Well, when I investigated for a piece I wrote for LisaBarger.com a few years ago I couldn't find any evidence that Sheryl Crow ever said any such thing. Sure, she did lots of *Ellen* interviews around the time this story first appeared and she did talk about her cancer in several of those segments.

But in no segment I could find did she ever blame a plastic water bottle for her disease.

I also pointed out that the amount of time your bottle of water spends in your car is probably only a fraction of its actual lifespan. After all, long before you take that bottle of water out on your next run, it's probably already spent days—if not weeks—in hot conditions.

- First it spent time in the bottler's warehouse waiting to be picked up. Then it was trucked in an un-refrigerated trailer.
- Next, it spent some time in a distribution center.
- Then it sat, most likely unrefrigerated, in your grocer's storage area.

When you think about it that way, does it really make sense to worry about "chemicals" leaching out after just a couple of hours in a hot car? I don't think so but if this is something that worries you, you could just resolve not to drink pre-packaged water.

And you could always just do what I did--buy yourself a reusable stainless steel water bottle and refill it as you need to.

"EAT LOCAL HONEY FOR SEASONAL ALLERGY."'

The logic behind this myth goes something like, "*If you get hay fever you should start eating locally produced honey because of the little bits of pollen that will be trapped in the honey. The tiny amounts of pollen will act like a vaccine and let your body get used to what you're allergic to.*"

It sounds like an interesting idea but there's (almost) no proof that it actually works. There's a lot of evidence, though, that pollen in honey can trigger allergic reactions in susceptible people. And in some cases, those reactions have been life-threatening.

Then there are also serious flaws in the idea that local honey would contain local allergens, anyway. There's simply no way to tell if the allergen you're allergic to is even in the honey without laboratory tests.

And even if it was, how could you possibly control the "dosage"? The idea is to consume only tiny amounts of the "bad" pollen, right? How could you possibly trust that the amount of pollen you were ingesting was tiny enough to stimulate and "re-train" your immune system and not cause a full-blown allergic reaction?

Consider also that bees don't generally make honey with typical allergy-causing plants. The pollen you're allergic to, say the experts I've consulted, would most likely be wind-carried and not bee-carried.

As for the actual scientific evidence . . . well there isn't much. A 2002 study from the University of Connecticut Health Center tested a variety of honeys on allergy suffers and found that none of the honeys--not even the raw, local stuff--did anything to ease allergy symptoms.

There is a little bit of good news, though. Honey does seem to affect the body's mast cells, which could, perhaps, mean fewer (or less severe) symptoms. But that suppressive effect is linked to the honey itself, and not any particular pollen.

And I did recently come across a study from Finland that looked at birch pollen honey as a potential treatment for birch allergy. In this study, which was small, the men and women who consumed birch tree honey for about 5 months did have fewer "allergy" days and less-severe symptoms than the study volunteers who consumed regular honey and did better even than the study's control group, which used only conventional allergy medications.

Will this new study convince skeptics that local honey is useful after all? I don't know but I have to admit I'll be interested to see if the results hold up.

Sources:

Rajan, T., et al. (2002). Effect of Ingestion of Honey on Symptoms of Rhinoconjunctivitis. *Annals of Allergy, Asthma & Immunology*.

Saarinen, K., et al. (2011). Birch Pollen Honey for Birch Pollen Allergy--A Randomized, Controlled Pilot Study. *International Archives of Allergy & Immunology*.

"WE'RE ALL MALNOURISHED BECAUSE OUR SOILS HAVE BEEN STRIPPED OF NUTRIENTS."

I'd heard this myth for years before I finally sat down to investigate it. According to believers, we're all malnourished these days because there are no natural nutrients left in our soils. Here's the 2010 piece that resulted from that investigation (with a follow-up below):

The Myth of Depleted Soils--Is It True?

How many times have you heard about how non-nutritious our fruits and vegetables are these days because of over-farming? According to the "depleted soils" myth, our croplands have been so damaged by years and years of mainstream farming that our foods are no longer nutritious enough to sustain us. They contain, some people claim, only a fraction of the vitamins and minerals the same fruits and vegetables contained 50 years ago.

And worst of all, these depletions are causing everything from worsened menopause symptoms to cancers that are striking younger and younger folks. It sounds scary but, as we'll show you, it's not true.

Consider these facts about the "depleted soils" myth:

- While it's true that minerals can be depleted by over-farming, there's absolutely no truth that crops deplete the soil of vitamins. Why? Because there are no vitamins in dirt in the first place. Growing plants don't absorb vitamins from soil—they make their own vitamins as they grow.

- Common sense would tell you that depleted soils simply wouldn't allow plants to produce fruits and vegetables in sizable numbers but our ability to grow more food crops per acre of land has leapfrogged in the past 40 years. In 1950, for example, the average acre of corn produced a little over 37 bushels of corn per acre; in 1992 that number had risen to nearly 129 bushels per acre.

- Many crop farms practice an ancient farming technique known as "rotation farming"--precisely to combat "over-farming". In rotation farming heavy-feeder crops are planted and harvested then the land is either allowed to sit for a time or is planted with crops that are specifically chosen to return nutrients back to the soil.

- Finally, as experts from the University of Wisconsin point out in their piece titled *"Are Depleted Soils Causing a Reduction in the Mineral Content Of Food Crops?"* farmers not only routinely test for things like mineral content; they also fertilize their fields regularly. How can a plot of land that's being regularly supplemented with minerals be mineral deficient?

Why does the "depleted soil" myth persist? Well, there has been some data suggesting that mineral contents are declining in some of the world's farmlands. But that data is controversial and some experts believe it's been taken out of context by people pushing their own political or environmental agendas.

So is there really any truth to the myth about depleted soils causing low-quality foods? Well, after looking at the facts, what do YOU think?

Source:

Lyne, J., Barak, P. (2000). Are Depleted Soils Causing a Reduction in the Mineral Content Of Food Crops? Accessible at soils.wisc.edu.

Tisdale, S., et al. (1992). Soil fertility and fertilizers; an introduction to nutrient management. Prentice Hall.

Rothman, M. (2002). Menopause: Myths vs. Facts. Accessed from fwhc.org May 26, 2010. (Claims depleted soils are worsening menopause.)

Cawood, M. (2009). Why depleted soils are making us sick. Accessed from theland.farmonline.com.au on May 26, 2010. (Claims depleted soils are increasing breast cancer in younger women.)

####

Shortly after I published this article at LisaBarger.com I began to get emails and web comments telling me I was wrong. A few of them pointed me to a 2004 study done by Donald Davis and published in the *Journal of the American College of Nutrition*. That study **did** find that some of our food crops are less nutrient-rich than they were a few decades ago.

If you look at what Davis actually says, though, he doesn't "credit" worsening soil or over-farming for the decline in some nutrients. He speculates that it's the crops themselves that are the problem. To quote Davis himself: "We conclude that the most likely explanation was changes in cultivated varieties used today compared to 50 years ago."

He goes on to say, ". . . when you select for yield, crops grow bigger and faster, but they don't necessarily have the ability to make or uptake nutrients at the same, faster rate."

You can read Davis' comments about his research--in context--here: http://www.utexas.edu/news/2004/12/01/nr_chemistry/

"COLLOIDAL SILVER IS AN ESSENTIAL MINERAL."

Colloidal silver is made by suspending tiny, tiny particles of real silver in some type of liquid--usually plain water. And while this odd-sounding concoction does appear to have some legitimate medical uses, it's nowhere the medical panacea its hawkers claim. Let's take a look at a 2005 article I wrote about the oral use of colloidal silver (and why virtually all the claims about oral silver are bunk) and then we'll look at a couple of studies that hint at its potential in treating jock itch and preventing post-dental-surgery infections:

Colloidal Silver - 2005 Article

Silver is an element that's used in a number of commercial products. Electronics, jewelry, photo processing and dentistry are just a few of the industries that use this precious metal. But silver—especially tiny particles of silver suspended in some sort of a vitamin-rich liquid supplement—has also gained popularity in "natural" medicine for its alleged ability to kill a variety of microorganisms in the body.

How Silver Is Used in Medicine

Silver has been used medicinally for centuries and is still used, albeit less frequently, even today. Silver nitrates, for example, are still used to prevent conjunctivitis in newborns. And silver sulfadizine is used in the treatments of burns. But it's important to know that these products are always applied topically—they're never ingested—and have documented side effects.

But colloidal silver is ingested. Colloidal silver is made by suspending extremely fine particles of silver in some sort of liquid. Some colloidal silver products have flavors, sweeteners and other additives, but, essentially, they're just silver particles and plain water. In addition to oral usage, colloidal silver products are sprayed onto the skin, sprayed into the nose or injected into a vein.

What Colloidal Silver Is Supposed To Do For You

Claims of colloidal silver's alleged health benefits abound. [A now-defunct website] makes the innocuous claim that colloidal silver can "help with diarrhea" while [another defunct website] goes a little further and lists "antibacterial", "non-toxic with no recorded side effects" and "flushing out toxins" among it's many claims. But perhaps the boldest claim about colloidal silver comes from Sharon Hubbs-Kreft's page at LocalHarvest.org. Hubbs-Kreft calls her brand of colloidal silver "a healing tincture" that "is almost a cure all" that no pharmaceutical antibiotic can match.

The TRUTH About Colloidal Silver

The truth is, silver—whether "colloidal" or not—serves no known nutritional function in the human body. It's not an essential mineral and doesn't need to be supplemented by taking expensive (and potentially dangerous) colloidal silver supplements.

And colloidal silver can have side effects like seizures, kidney damage, and skin irritation. In very large doses, it can also cause a harmless but irreversible skin discoloration known as argyria.

Additionally, colloidal silver can interfere with your body's ability to absorb certain types of medications.

These are only a few of the reasons why, in 1999, the FDA issued a ruling stating that no colloidal silver products are considered "safe" or "effective". In the years since, both the FDA and FTC have issued numerous warnings to companies hawking colloidal silver products via web sites, brochures and flyers.

"But Silver Is Used in Water Filters!"

Yes. Silver (not "colloidal" silver) is used in water filters to kill microorganisms and it does a good job at it. But there's a big difference between putting a germ in direct contact with silver (by forcing the water it's in through a water filter) and taking colloidal silver in the hopes that the silver particle will somehow find a foreign invader and destroy it. Currently, no legitimate scientific data exists to support the idea that colloidal silver works that way in the human body.

The bottom line on colloidal silver is that its use just isn't supported by science. And if you're pregnant, nursing, or treating a child with colloidal silver, it's absolutely vital that you discuss your colloidal silver use with a qualified medical professional before continuing, urge doctors.

Does that make it a scam? You tell me.

Despite the FDA's Final Rule on colloidal silver, it's still widely touted, especially on the internet. Just look at this 2009 Q&A from LisaBarger.com:

Is Colloidal Silver FDA-Approved? - Q&A

"How can you call colloidal silver a scam when this article [on a content farm website] PROVES the FDA approves of it?"

My answer: The author of that piece, [author's name has been removed], is incorrect. Colloidal silver is still considered an "unapproved drug" by the FDA and must be marketed without any health claims attached to it.

In 1999, in response to requests from various manufacturers and colloidal silver users, the FDA issued what is known as a "Final Rule". This ruling, effective September 16, 1999, stated that all over-the-counter colloidal silver products were to be officially recognized as "misbranded".

This ruling came about as the result of a 1996 proposal to classify colloidal silver as "not generally recognized as safe and effective". After 3 years of conversations with users, distributors and manufacturers, the FDA found insufficient evidence that colloidal silver was effective for any medical condition. The 1999 Final Rule made it official.

Perhaps the author of that piece is confusing colloidal silver, which is a liquid with tiny particles of silver suspended in it, with legitimate silver products which are medically used and recognized scientifically as effective for their various purposes.

Remember, there's a very big difference between putting silver into direct contact with a wound and taking a tablespoon of a "dissolved" silver potion and expecting it to somehow seek out all the bad germs in your body.

References:

Federal Register. (2009). Retrieved from: http://www.fda.gov/OHRMS/DOCKETS/98fr/081799a.pdf, March 30, 2009.

Weisenfelder, H. (2009). Colloidal Silver: An Alternative to Antibiotics. Retrieved from www.brighthub.com March 30.

####

Now, it probably sounds as though I was on a mission to rid the world of magic potions. But in 2009 I found a couple of studies that suggested that colloidal silver might just have some legit uses after all--at least when used topically. Here's the Q&A in which I cite those studies:

Colloidal Silver For Jock Itch & Athlete's Foot

In 2009 I answered this question in a Q&A at LisaBarger.com: *"I read on a forum about a guy who bathed his nether-regions with colloidal silver to cure jock itch. I know you're a skeptic when it comes to drinking the stuff but since it used to be used as an antibiotic, what do you think about using it this way?"*

Here's my answer:

That's a very interesting question and I agree with you. There's absolutely no scientific evidence that drinking colloidal silver can cure any infection, despite claims made on various web sites, forums and blogs, but the idea of using it topically may just have some merit.

I did run across a very interesting study from China. In 2008, a group of dental patients were divided into two groups during their dental extractions. One group had colloidal silver sponges inserted into their sockets while the other group did not. The rate of post-surgery "complications" in the silver group was a third of that of the non-treated group.

I'm not sure how relevant that actually is, but it might be something to think about.

I did actually find another study from China—this one published in 2009—that seemed to prove that colloidal preparations of silver had some anti-fungal actions. This was an *in vitro* study and not a study in real, living humans but, again, it may be something to think about.

So, does topically-applied colloidal silver really kill jock itch? Science doesn't yet say, "Yes," but it's a very interesting question.

References:

Cai, Y., et al. (2008). A clinical study of gelatamp colloidal silver gelatin sponge on preventing the complication of teeth extraction. *West China Journal of Stomatology.*

Bo. L., et al. (2009). A simple and 'green' synthesis of polymer-based silver colloids and their antibacterial properties. *Chemistry & Biodiversity.*

####

2009 was also the year we were all watching a big swine flu outbreak and wondering how bad it would really get. Here's a piece from that summer I wrote about colloidal silver sellers peddling it for swine flu:

Colloidal Silver For Swine Flu - Q&A

"Do you think colloidal silver can really cure swine flu?"

No, I don't think [the evidence shows that] colloidal silver will treat or cure the H1N1 virus. Remember, there's a very big difference between putting silver, which has legitimate medical uses, directly onto an infection and drinking minute bits of ground up silver in the hopes that those particles will somehow travel through your body and seek out a germ.

I'm really sorry that the manufacturers of this sham product have chosen to prey on the fears of the public by promoting this nonsense. Putting silver on the site of a bacterial infection goes back decades and it works. In fact, silver is still in use today for things like burns. And a few new studies published in legitimate medical journals even suggest that silver may help fight athlete's foot and the infection that sometimes develops after certain dental procedures.

BUT ... there has never been even one double-blind study that proved drinking the stuff did anything positive. Yes, silver can kill germs. But drinking tiny amounts of silver in the hopes that it will travel through your blood, seek out a germ and then destroy it is just wishful thinking.

Oh, and the guy everyone's buzzing about? The truth is Dr. [Name Removed]—the guy you see quoted all the time on those pro-silver web sites and blogs—has an honorary degree. He has, to my knowledge, never published any of his research in a single peer-reviewed journal. He works as a "full-time consultant" for a . . . want to guess or should I just tell you? He works as a consultant for a company that manufactures supplements.

Rather than depend on unproven and very expensive miracle cures like colloidal silver, your doctor might prefer you work toward strengthening your immune system naturally and focus on proven infection prevention methods like handwashing.

I did have to give colloidal silver a bit of quarter, though, when I answered this question about its use for conjunctivitis in 2010:

Colloidal Silver For Pink Eye --Does It Work? - Q&A

"Some people [on internet forums] are saying to wash your eyes with colloidal silver to cure pink eye. Does that really work?"

My answer: We can't actually give you medical advice but what we can tell you is that while colloidal silver may not be the miracle cure some of its users are claiming it is, there just might be some truth to this one. Under the supervision of a medical professional, colloidal silver might be helpful in some cases of bacterial conjunctivitis, or "pink eye".

There's absolutely no evidence—not even in "alternative" medical journals—to suggest that drinking colloidal silver does anything to fight any known infection. There are scores of websites, blogs and internet forums out there claiming otherwise, but there's just no scientific evidence to support their claims.

There are, however, a handful of studies suggesting that using colloidal silver on certain topical infections like athlete's foot might help control the infection. No one is suggesting that it can replace actual medications but there does seem to be at least a little bit of evidence that supports the use of colloidal silver in this way.

So could colloidal silver also help with an eye infection like "pink eye"? Well, although it wasn't actually "colloidal", silver was once widely used to cure STD-related conjunctivitis in newborns and various silver preparations were used well up into the 1940s as wound dressings.

And silver is still used medically today, even if it's been mostly replaced by pharmaceutical antibiotics. Burn victims are still often dressed with silver-impregnated bandages and silver is sometimes used in water filters to kill pathogens.

Does this mean we'd recommend colloidal silver for use with "pink eye"? We'll not go quite that far just yet but even we have to admit that the idea is intriguing.

Sources:

Brentano, L., et al. (1966). Antibacterial efficacy of a colloidal silver complex. *Surgical Forum*.

Bielefeldt, A., et al. (2009). Bacterial treatment effectiveness of point-of-use ceramic water filters. *Water Research*.

Schneider, G. (1984). Silver nitrate prophylaxis. *Canadian Medical Association Journal*.

Bo. L., et al. (2009). A simple and 'green' synthesis of polymer-based silver colloids and their antibacterial properties. *Chemistry & Biodiversity*.

####

Despite a few potentially positive studies on colloidal silver it's unlikely, in my opinion, that the US Food and Drug Administration, or FDA, will ever allow it to be sold with such health claims attached. And it's not just the fact that the FDA gets its hackles up at "alternative" medicine. This study I covered in 2010 didn't even look at colloidal silver but found that silver can accumulate in the body:

Silver Nanoparticles Linked to Liver Damage

A new study says that nanoparticles of silver from water filters, kitchen utensils and even our bedding and towels can accumulate in our bodies and cause minimal (but still measurable) damage to our livers.

In the past, silver has been widely regarded as inert in the body. Basically any "dose" under what would be required to cause argyria ("bluing" of the skin) was generally classified as non-toxic.

However, this doesn't seem to be entirely true. In this study laboratory animals were given specific "doses" of silver and then followed for several weeks. And what the researchers discovered after examining the animals at the end of the study was that these nanoparticles do accumulate in bodily organs—especially the kidneys and liver.

Why is this study a big deal? Well, silver can be added to everything from shampoos to bacteria-fighting sheets and towels. It's even found in some of those screw-on water filters that so many of us have. (It's also still used medically but that use is waning as better antibiotics come along.)

And believe it or not, there hasn't been a lot of study on just how all this silver exposure can affect us. Scientists have long known that we can consume or inhale tiny particles of silver from those types of germ-fighting products but very few studies have ever looked at the potential health effects of that exposure.

While this study didn't look specifically at any of the so-called "colloidal" silver products being marketed by some alternative health experts it does suggest that we may not know all we need to know about such preparations.

Source:

Kim, Y., et la. (2010). Subchronic oral toxicity of silver nanoparticles. *Particle and Fibre Toxicology.*

####

This study actually came after the FDA issued a formal request to all US healthcare professionals, asking them to warn their patients about the potential dangers of consuming colloidal silver:

FDA Again Cautions Health Professionals About "Colloidal" Silver - News Article

The U.S. Food & Drug Administration, or FDA, is once again asking healthcare professionals to caution patients about the dangers of a popular alternative "medicine" known as colloidal silver.

In medicine, silver has legitimate medical purposes. It is still used, for example, to prevent eye infections in newborns and to kill germs in bandages and wound dressings. Taken internally, though, silver serves no known purpose. It is considered a nonessential mineral and has never been shown to treat, cure or prevent any disease when consumed in its "colloidal" form.

But internal use of silver does have a very real side effect known as argyria. This harmless but permanent discoloration of the skin has been documented in at least 70 Americans. Experts aren't sure exactly how silver causes argyria but they believe that it binds to proteins. This may also explain why argyria patients often get even darker when their skin is exposed to sunlight.

The FDA urges anyone who has been affected to report their experiences to the FDA's MedWatch program. And, of course, they also urge any consumer considering taking colloidal silver to discuss their use with a licensed health care professional before doing so.

Source:

U.S. Food & Drug Administration. (2009). Letter to Health Care Professionals: FDA Consumer Advisory Regarding Dietary Supplements that Contain Silver.

####

Hardcore believers in colloidal silver won't be swayed by the opinions of the FDA, of course, but they might listen to their own gurus. Two of the most prominent promoters of "natural" health, Ray Sahelian and Andrew Weil, have both addressed colloidal silver with their own audiences.

Sahelian called silver "worth a try" but admitted that he found it "difficult" while Weil was a bit more blunt. He called the claims about colloidal silver "nonsense" and "unproven" and added that colloidal silver is not a substitute for antibiotics.

"WE ARE ALL DEHYDRATED AND NOTHING BUT PURE WATER WILL REHYDRATE YOU."

Of all the "natural" health myths I've tackled, this one has been among the most stubborn. The myth goes something along these lines, "Every person is walking around in a chronic state of mild dehydration because no one drinks enough water anymore. Mild dehydration is why you're having headaches, eczema and digestion problems. It's also why you're always tired, why you're fat and why you can't concentrate at work."

The myth then usually goes on to say that only pure water will rehydrate you. Some "experts" will allow a bit of herbal tea but coffee and sodas are definitely on the "don't drink" list. Don't even think about prepackaged energy drinks or an evening cocktail.

The truth is, the scientific evidence says that most of that is complete bunk. Yes, it's true that alcoholic beverages will dehydrate you and it's true that caffeine acts as a diuretic. BUT to then go on and say that we're all chronically dehydrated and that only pure water will fix it? That's complete nonsense.

So how can caffeinated coffee act as a diuretic but also hydrate you? The answer is simple--the water you get from a cup of coffee is greater than the water you lose to the caffeine.

One of the most famous studies to prove this was a 2003 study done at the University of Nebraska's Center for Human Nutrition. In that study, researchers recruited a group of men and divided them into 2 groups. For 3 days the men in 1 group ate normally but drank only plain water. The men in the other group ate normally but drank beverages other than plain water. Everything the men ate, drank and did was documented.

When researchers analyzed the men's test results, they found absolutely no difference between the men who drank nothing but water and the men who drank no water at all for 3 days. Nothing used as a marker for hydration was different.

OK, but what about looking just at caffeine? Surely that's not safe for athletes, right?

Well, as it turns out, the evidence says otherwise. Another 2003 study--this one from the University of Washington's Department of Family Medicine-- looked at caffeine use in athletes and found that it improved athletic performance and endurance while having no significant effect on either overall hydration levels or the body's electrolyte balance.

But let's get back to the plain old folks who aren't out there running a 5K every day. Surely the average American drinks far too much coffee, right? Well, only your doctor can tell you how much (if any) coffee or tea is appropriate for you but I've covered medical studies that looked at people who drank 6 or more cups of coffee a day and I've never seen mentions of those people being dehydrated.

And as far as the claims that we're all walking around mildly dehydrated goes . . . well, a 2012 feature piece in *BMJ* alleges that at least some of the credit for that myth goes to the companies that make sports drinks.

Remember, as recently as the early 1970s long-distance runners were actually advised NOT to "pre-hydrate" before a race or to over-hydrate during a race for fear that it would slow them down while providing no benefit.

But then, beverage companies began touting "sports drinks" and suddenly, everyone was supposedly dehydrated. In fact, claims the *BMJ* piece, the entire idea of hydration science was cooked up by scientists on beverage companies' payrolls. Their "guidelines"--and a good bit of fear mongering-- eventually filtered down to the normal, everyday consumer, convincing us that chronic mild dehydration is a common problem.

So what about the old 8-glasses-a-day advice? Well, that one was tackled by Dr. Spero Tsindo in a 2012 issue of *Australian and New Zealand Journal of Public Health*. In that editorial Tsindo points out that drinking large volumes of any beverage at once is just wasteful. Your body, says Tsindo, can only process a certain volume of liquid at once. Drink a lot of any beverage and most of it will be lost in your urine before your body even gets a chance to use it.

"MANUKA HONEY CURES IT."

The oldest medical study on manuka honey that I can find only goes back to 1991 but it wasn't until the mid-2000s or so that manuka honey's popularity seemed to explode here in the US. But as amazing and as promising as manuka honey is, is it really the cure-all its sellers often claim? As it turns out, manuka is showing tremendous promise but it's not the only honey to do so. And in many cases, it's not even the most effective.

But before I get into why manuka honey may not be worth your money, let's look at exactly what it is. Here's a 2008 piece I wrote on it for LisaBarger.com:

Manuka Honey--Is It A Scam - Q&A

Question: *"What do you think about manuka honey? Is it a scam?"*

My answer: Produced almost exclusively in New Zealand, manuka honey is really just plain old honey made by plain old honeybees. The only difference is that this honey is made from the pollen of the manuka bush.

Manuka is known botanically as *Leptospermum scoparium* and is a perennial shrub or small tree. It's found mainly in New Zealand but, contrary to what you'll read on some pro-manuka blogs, the tree is also found in various parts of Australia.

It's sometimes referred to as "tea tree" and it is, in fact, related to the "true" tea tree, *Melaleuca alternifolia*.

What Manuka Is Supposed To Do For You

As is always the case with a new "miracle cure", exaggerated claims and absurd stories of miraculous healing are common. Testimonials and sales spiels are found around the 'net, including at least one on Amazon.com, proclaiming manuka honey "a miracle". It's also said to give "astounding results" and has even convinced one UK resident identified only as "Ms. M" that it saved her life.

What Science Says About All This

Excited testimonials found on sites hawking honey are one thing but scientific proof of this honey's effectiveness are something else. And, actually, manuka honey seems to be standing up quite nicely to scientific study. A 2008 study published in *International Wound Journal* found that by lowering the pH of skin wounds, manuka honey encouraged healing. Researchers were quick to note that more research should be done before honey becomes a cure-all for wounds but this study seems promising.

But Is It Really The Honey? Or Is It The Bees?

Manuka believers have long claimed that this type of honey contains a special antibacterial compound they refer to as the "Unique Manuka Factor" or UMF.

If that sounds a little "out there", take heart. The "unique factor" is actually a substance known to chemists as methylglyoxal. And while methylglyoxal does seem to be the "active" ingredient in manuka, it is by no means the only "active" component. A 2007 study published in the *Polish Journal of Microbiology* identified even more types of honey with potent anti-microbial actions. And some of those honeys rival (and perhaps even surpass) the anti-microbial actions of manuka.

Lisa's Opinion

Ultimately, I see absolutely nothing wrong with "designer" honeys, other than the fact that they're expensive. Some of the research is extremely promising. But it's important to remember that much of what you see on the internet is commercially-motivated and many of the people behind those claims may exaggerate or even lie about scientific evidence to fit a money-driven agenda. As with all other "miracle" cures, if it sounds too good to be true, it probably is.

Sources:

Australian National Botanic Gardens. (1996). Leptospermum scoparium.

Amazon.com. (2007). Retrieved from amazon.com/Manuka-Honey-Active-Certified-1-Pound/dp/B000P3JJAO on May 29, 2008.

PR-Inside.com. (2008). Retrieved from pr-inside.com/print606453.htm on May 29, 2008.

Nature's Nectar Limited. (No Date). Retrieved from manukahoney.co.uk/Fact%20Sheet.pdf on May 29, 2008.

Gethin, G. (2008). The impact of Manuka honey dressings on the surface pH of chronic wounds. *International Wound Journal.*

Mavric, E., et al. (2008). Identification and quantification of methylglyoxal as the dominant antibacterial constituent of Manuka (Leptospermum scoparium) honeys from New Zealand. *Molecular Nutrition & Food Research.*

Temaru, E., et al. (2007). Antibacterial activity of honey from stingless honeybees (Hymenoptera; Apidae; Meliponinae). *Polish Journal of Microbiology.*

####

It wasn't long, of course, before other producers of exotic honeys began to elbow their honeys into the public eyes. Here's a news piece I did just about a year later:

Manuka Honey Isn't All That, After All - News Article

If you follow "natural" medicine at all, you've seen glowing articles about a new "designer" honey on the market called manuka. Manuka believers claim it's a cure for just about anything that ails you, including ulcers, burns and antibiotic-resistant infections. But a new study says that as amazing as manuka honey may be, it's not all that different from others.

It is believed that all raw honeys have at least some antibacterial properties, especially when applied topically. Researchers in Malaysia wanted to see just how well their honey, tualang honey, stood up against manuka's proven germ-killing actions so they used different concentrations of a "honey broth" against 13 different germs.

What they found was that tualang honey, which is made from the nectar of the tualang tree, or *Koompassia excelsa*, is every bit as good as the more expensive (and more hyped) manuka. Against some pathogens manuka did a little better and against other strains tualang performed better. But all-in-all, the differences were minor.

Perhaps we would do well to stop marveling at any particular honey and start thinking just a little bit more about the tiny little creatures who produce this bounty for us—the bees.

Source:

Tan, H., et al. (2009). The antibacterial properties of Malaysian tualang honey against wound and enteric microorganisms in comparison to manuka honey. Provisional PDF accessed from biomedcentral.com September 16, 2009.

####

Then there was this piece--on a honey produced in Chile:

Ulmo Honey Legit Competitor to Other Honeys, Says Study

A new study says that a type of honey produced mainly in Chile is actually more effective at killing the MRSA germ than manuka honey and it's equally effective at killing other potentially dangerous germs, too.

MRSA, or Methicillin-resistant *Staphylococcus aureus*, is a type of staph infection that has become so resistant to pharmaceutical antibiotics that it can be almost impossible to cure once the bacteria set up shop in a human being.

While a growing number of us have MRSA living harmlessly in the mucus layer of our noses, for example, the MRSA can be deadly if it travels to other areas of the body. And, yes, this is the so-called "flesh-eating bacteria" that made so much news a few years ago.

Naturally, health experts have been searching for new ways to both prevent these infections and cure them once they present themselves. Honey, which has potent anti-microbial abilities, has been the focus of much of that research and many people have heard of the "miracle" honeys like manuka.

But while manuka may have been the first of the "designer" honeys to hit it big here in the US, it's not the only one and it certainly isn't the most effective. Now, scientists say that ulmo honey—a honey produced by our South American neighbors—is actually better at killing MRSA.

The ulmo tree is known botanically as *Eucryphia cordifolia* and grows throughout Argentina and Chile. In recent years it's also been extensively cultivated as an ornamental along the Pacific coast of the U.S. In its natural habitat the tree is highly prized for its hard, decay-resistant wood and highly scented blossoms.

Source:

Sherlock, O., et al. (2010). Comparison of the antimicrobial activity of Ulmo honey from Chile and Manuka honey against methicillin-resistant Staphylococcus aureus, Escherichia coli and Pseudomonas aeruginos. *BMC Complementary and Alternative Medicine.*

#####

And then there was this one--also from 2010--on honey made from plain old honeydew nectar:

Honeydew Honey More Effective Than Manuka

If you're even a casual student of "natural" health you've probably heard of a new "designer" honey called manuka. It burst onto the alternative medicine scene a few years ago and some of its proponents have been making some pretty amazing claims about it.

Actual scientific research, unfortunately, hasn't been as kind to it. Several recent studies have found that other varieties of honey were actually more effective at killing germs than this new miracle.

And, now, a study from Slovakia drives yet another nail into manuka's coffin of exclusive claims. In this study researchers from that country's

Institute of Zoology and the Slovak Medical University tested manuka honey against honey made from honeydew nectar and found that when it came to killing a nasty infection called *Stenotrophomonas maltophilia* plain old honeydew honey actually worked better—even when the germ was resistant to standard hospital antibiotic drugs.

Honeydew is a type of muskmelon; it's known botanically as *Cucumis melo*. Honeydew happens to be a type known as a "smooth-skinned" melon and its cultivar name is White Antibes. These days honeydew melons are grown around the world, both commercially and in backyard gardens of all sizes.

The germ the honeydew honey was tested against is a germ that can be very difficult to treat, especially in people who have weakened immune systems. In particular, it can be a real issue for folks who have breathing or feeding tubes and can also exist quite happily in I.V. lines.

For this study researchers took 20 resistant strains of the germ from cancer patients and tested both honeydew honey and manuka honey against them. What they found was that the honeydew honey worked better on 16 of the 20 strains tested.

Source:

Majtan, J., et al. (2010). Honeydew honey as a potent antibacterial agent in eradication of multi-drug resistant Stenotrophomonas maltophilia isolates from cancer patients. *Phytotherapy Research.*

I wrote those news pieces not to detract in any way from manuka honey but to point out that you have a choice. Honey is amazing stuff but you don't have to pay $40 a jar to get the potential health benefits.

"DOCTORS DON'T KNOW ANYTHING ABOUT HERBS—AND THEY DON'T WANT TO."

Some of the most divisive and hurtful myths in alternative and "natural" medicine are about how doctors don't, can't or won't recommend herbal remedies because they're too ignorant, too biased or on the "Big Pharma" payroll.

The truth is some doctors **are** completely closed to the idea of "herbal" medicine. (I actually did have a physician roll his eyes at me once.) And some doctors won't recommend herbs because they already have safe, effective pharmaceutical remedies they trust.

But the vast majority of doctors I have spoken to in my career were at least willing to entertain the idea of "alternative" treatments--so long as those treatments are already proven safe and effective. Doctors--whether they work in mainstream medicine or alternative medicine--are a diverse group of people.

OK, you may be thinking, so what about all the money doctors won't make by prescribing herbal remedies?

Consider this: In 2012 Americans spent more than $594,000,000 on herbal remedies and nutritional supplements. And that doesn't include products like "herbal" cosmetics or herbal teas. Half a billion dollars is a lot of money for doctors to just turn their backs on, don't you think?

Does it really make sense to accuse doctors of being greedy and taking kickbacks from pharmaceutical companies when they could just as easily get those kickbacks from "natural" drug companies?

You may have also heard that doctors won't prescribe herbs because they aren't patentable medicines. To that, I say, "Look at Metamucil®." It's an "herbal" product—after all, its main ingredient is psyllium. And it's not patented but the folks who make it are certainly doing all right with it.

Obviously, a patent isn't necessary for a "natural" medicine to be commercially successful.

So what about the idea that doctors don't know enough about herbs to use them confidently? There may be some truth to that but that's changing. Most medical schools in the US are doing at least something to educate medical students about non-mainstream therapies.

And as for older doctors . . . well, they've always had access to research on herbal remedies. There are research papers on herbal remedies and alternative therapies published every year--and they're not just in "fringe" journals that only marginalized crackpots read, either.

Those studies are peer-reviewed and published in major medical journals like *JAMA* and the *New England Journal of Medicine*.

"THANKS" & SOME CLOSING THOUGHTS

You might think from reading *10 Lies Your Herbalist Told You* that I hate alternative medicine and the people who practice it.

I don't.

I may not have the title "Herbalist" next to my name anymore but I do still run more than a dozen websites devoted to the science of herbal remedies, natural health and alternative therapies. I just believe that if you're going to say, "Buy my stuff," you should be able to give people more than vague explanations and a cutesy lesson in folk medicine.

If you agree, please check out more of my work at your favorite bookseller.

And "Thank you!" for reading.

ABOUT THE AUTHOR

Lisa Barger has been called "one of our greatest educators in the alternative medicine field" and someone who is "on a mission" to debunk myths and scams with a "pit bull energy".

She is the founder of, and principle writer for, the LisaBarger.com family of websites, covering food safety, natural health scams, infant product recalls and   more.

Her columns are syndicated through the Amazon's Kindle Blogs program.

Lisa currently lives in Cabot, Arkansas.

www.ingramcontent.com/pod-product-compliance
Lightning Source LLC
Chambersburg PA
CBHW030538290526
45786CB00004B/1763